VEGAN PROTEIN YOGA SMOOTHIES

Contains 50 Smoothie Recipes to
Build a STRONG and HEALTHY
Body from the Inside Out

Mariana Correa
Certified Sports Nutritionist

Copyright Page

2015 Vegan Protein Yoga Smoothies

ISBN:1523960809

Acknowledgement

To my father, I admire your dedication and hard work and continue to learn from you every day.

About the author

Mariana Correa is a certified sports nutritionist and former professional tennis player.
Mariana reached a career high of 26 in the world in juniors with wins over Anna Ivanovich (former #1 WTA in the world) and many other top 100 WTA players.

She competed successfully all over the world in over 26 countries and hundreds of cities including in London for Wimbledon, Paris for the French Open and in Australia for the world championships. She also represented Ecuador in Fed Cup, where the team reached the finals in their group.

During her career she was awarded the fair play award many times, proving to be not only an excellent player, but also a role model for other athletes.

Being an athlete herself she understands what it takes to be the best in what you love.

Mariana is a certified sports nutritionist with years of experience in proper nutrition and hydration for high performance athletes.

She combines her love and knowledge in sports and nutrition in this book to provide you with all the information you need to succeed.

Description

Supercharge your yoga lifestyle with healthy and delicious vegan protein smoothies. Whether you're looking for a meal replacement smoothie, a breakfast smoothie, a smoothie for before or after your workout you'll have 50 smoothie recipes to choose from. These are the best vegan protein shakes for any yogi who is looking to:

- Feel Healthier
- Increase Energy Levels
- Enhance your Performance

Build a strong and healthy body from the inside out. You will enhance your performance by drinking all the nutrients your body needs. A healthy nutrition is the foundation of your training program and athletic development.

This book includes tips on healthy nutrition, proper hydration, the organic diet and 50 easy vegan recipes that will set you on the path of your best yoga practice.

The author Mariana Correa is a former professional athlete and certified sports nutritionist that competed successfully all over the world. She shares years of experience both as an athlete and a coach bringing a priceless perspective.

Table of Contents

Introduction

Achieve your Best Poses

"Most people have no idea how amazing their body is designed to perform" Mariana Correa

Most people believe being vegan means eating nothing but lettuce and tomatoes. At first they try eating only broccoli one day, then only carrots the next. By day three their goals and diet are out the door. With this book you will learn there is so much more to a vegan diet than carrots and broccoli.

There is such a great variety in a vegan diet and you don't need to be a professional chef to achieve your goals either. In our last chapter you will find 50 great recipes for yogis that are simple, affordable and easy to prepare.

 Let's begin by understanding your body is perfection. Yes, no matter what you think it's perfect. Every single cell works together in synchronicity allowing you to be healthy and perform your everyday activities and training.

Do you have any idea of all the cells that are working together in order for you to read this book or something as simple as the process of breathing? Your body is incredible, but in order to stay in top shape it needs your help.

An active lifestyle combined with good nutrition is the best way to stay healthy.

Nutrition is eighty percent habit. You most likely have had the same nutritional habits for years and years. It will take time, discipline and constant support to change your habits and reach your potential.

Yes, it's absolutely necessary to have a great training program and without it you won't accomplish much, but any champion can tell you that the single most important factor in creating the ultimate body is a proper nutrition plan.

There is only enough room at the top for the ones who really want it.

Nothing will ever come for free or granted. Do you love it enough to fight day in and out to reach your goals?

Yes! Wonderful, then let's get started.

Chapter 1
All about Protein

Protein comes from the word Primary in Greek. You must consider it as a 'Primary' addition to your everyday meals in order to achieve your goals.Protein functions in the body as a primary building block for muscle, skin, hair and several other tissues.

Protein is so important in our bodies, that after water has been excluded seventy five percent of your body weight that is left is made of protein.

Protein is similar to building blocks in our bodies called amino acids, these are connected together in diverse patterns to form specific proteins with diverse characteristics. Over twenty different amino acids exist, of these amino acids eight are determined to be vital because they cannot be produced by the body but are essential for survival. The body uses amino acids transiting in the blood stream, released from the breakdown of tissues, or eaten in the diet to make protein.

Protein varies from carbohydrate and fat, being that the body rarely stores protein, hence it is crucial in your diet.

The importance of protein for a yogi is for several reasons:

Protein has many important roles in the body including the composition of enzymes; which are imperative proteins that help responses occur in the body, such as releasing from the food we eat. Proteins also have the task to transport proteins such as hemoglobin; which is an iron comprising protein that transports oxygen to active muscles via the bloodstream.

Protein is the only nutrient directly in charge for building muscle. By being a straight originator to building muscle protein is indispensable for muscle recovery and growth.

This is the main reason we are focusing so much on protein for yogis. Every time you exercise your muscles are strained and must be renovated, protein assists in this process.

Many believe the main source for protein in through animal meat, but as you will read in this book, this couldn't be further from the truth.

In the athletic world many think that a plant based diet can't provide enough protein for a high performance level. Nutritionists have now demonstrated through various studies that this is not true. Athletes can consume enough vegetables, and hemp seeds, quinoa, beans, nuts, and more to acquire the protein required.

Studies have also demonstrated that a plant based diet can help reduce your risk of diabetes, cancer and heart disease. It also allows for quicker recovery from exercising and injuries by improving blood and oxygen flow.

By maintaining a vegan diet you will eliminate many processed foods that enhance inflammation in the body and will decrease performance.

Chapter 2

Vegan Enlightened

The first question that needs to be answered is what exactly it means to be on a vegan diet.

Vegans do not eat meat, fish or poultry. In addition to this, vegans do not use any animal products or by-products such as dairy products, leather, fur, silk, wool, cosmetics, eggs or anything derived from animal products. So in conclusion, unless it's plant derived, it's a no-go.

Why exactly do vegans adapt to these conditions? There are many reasons why vegans make this choice :

- The main aim why many chose veganism is due to moral reasons. By consuming animal products one is inevitably contributing to the demeaning conditions in which most animals spend their lives before being consumed.

- Another reason for veganism is health. Vegan diets are diverse, with richness in fresh, colorful and nutrient dense foods. Which promote overall better health as well as an enhanced performance for athletes.

- Others simply do not enjoy the taste of meat or animal products such as milk or eggs.

Whatever your reasons are this book will guide you in the right direction. People who make the switch from a normal diet to a vegan diet will see big changes right away. This will sound very appealing to those with health issues. For example if you have high blood pressure, this will decrease; if you're overweight you may shed those unwanted pounds quicker.

The best way to succeed in this diet is to understand that at the beginning this transition will not be easy. The road to a healthy lifestyle is paved with many temptations. It helps to have a support group, friends or family who will help you along the way.

Another key to success is to do your homework. Make sure you read the labels on the products you consume and use to make sure they are vegan.

Vegan History, How it all Began

The beginning of veganism has a foundation as early as the 1800s around the world. But officially in the U.S.A. the concept began as early as 1944 in North America, but it wasn't until 1949 when Leslie J Cross properly defined veganism. The concept began as a simple concept as "The principle of the emancipation of animals from exploitation by man."

Ultimately the definition of veganism was further illuminated by the American Vegan Society in 1979 as:

"A philosophy and way of living which seeks to exclude- as far as is possible and practicable- all forms of exploitation of, and cruelty to, animals for food, clothing or any other purpose; and by extension, promoted the development and use of animal-free alternatives for the benefit of humans, animals and the environment. In dietary terms it denotes the practice of dispensing with all products derived wholly or partly from animals."

Fast forwarding to this day and age this concept has remained true to vegans all around the world. There is a greater availability of vegan foods at supermarkets allowing for even more variety in the vegan diet.

In the following chapter we will discuss in depth what can be consumed in the vegan diet.

Chapter 3

Vegan Foods

"You don't have to be great to start, but you have to start to be great." Zig Ziglar

Most people have the misconception all they can eat is lettuce and tofu as a vegan, which comes as a surprise to me in this day and age with the wealth of information available.

The vegan diet consists of only plant-derived foods. This doesn't mean you'll be breaking the bank or eating fancier meals. The most inexpensive and nutritious vegan foods can be found all around you, from your backyard, the farmers market and your local supermarket. From fresh produce, grains, legumes, fruits, nuts and seeds to now available vegan cheeses, desserts, veggie burgers and much more.

A healthy and balanced vegan diet contains these food groups:

1. Grains
2. Vegetables

3. Fruits
4. Legumes, Seeds and Nuts

The amounts and combinations of each of these mentioned here will serve as a blueprint since each individual is unique the precise amounts for each will vary according to age, weight, health conditions, and nutrient and energy requirements.

1. Grains- these provide us with fiber, minerals, proteins, and antioxidants. Our goal is to consume mostly intact whole grains such as oats, brown rice, and millet. The amount of daily servings varies on your individual needs.

2. Vegetables- these are a huge part of the vegan diet. By consuming a wide variety of vegetables you can make sure your body will be receiving an assortment of necessary vitamins and minerals.

3. Fruits – these provide us with fiber, vitamins and a vast amount of antioxidants. Ideally we get a full

amount of vitamins from fresh fruits instead of fruit juices or frozen fruits.

4. Legumes, Seeds and Nuts – a vast amount of the daily required amount of protein will become available in this food group. This group includes legumes such as split peas, beans, lentils, and more. It also includes seeds such as sunflower seeds, pumpkin seeds, quinoa, and more.

In addition to this vegans can consume many foods that many others are familiar with. Such as hot dogs, burgers, ice cream, and cheese. These familiar foods have been adapted to a vegan diet by substituting animal products with alternatives such as a veggie burger, a coconut ice cream, a vegan hot dog and many more.

Vegans enjoy many of the same foods as other diets do, such as chips and salsa, pasta, and most breads are also vegan.

For many these changes can be tough at the beginning, but with simple substitutions you can easily switch to a vegan diet. Let's see some simple substitutions that can help you with this transition:

Cow's milk is probably one of the easiest to substitute with so many plant based alternatives now available in the supermarkets.

- Soy milk is extremely healthy and some brands will even fortify it with protein and vitamin D.

- Rice milk is made from the liquid of crushed rice with a light taste and contains similar amounts of calcium as cow's milk.

- Almond Milk this milk is ideal for desserts and baking, is high in healthy fats.

- Oat Milk contains a high amount of fiber and iron and is very easy to make. By simply leaving rolled oats soaking in water overnight, blend, strain and voila.

- Coconut Milk is low in calcium and in calories but still packs in protein, vitamins and minerals. Creamer texture allows for creamy sauces and desserts.

Cheese: Companies that make our milk alternatives also tend to make cheese and yogurt from these milks. You can find an interesting variety of cheeses for melting or ricotta or cottage cheese with these milks as well.
- Soy cheese is specially a great alternative as it melts and tastes just like cow's milk.

Eggs: There are many alternatives for eggs, depending on what kind of meal you're preparing, whether it's sweet or salty you have many options. Among these are:

- Apple sauce is a creative alternative, with only ¼ cup needed to replace one egg.

- Ground Flax seeds will provide you with a healthy amount of Omega-3 fats and fiber. I would recommend this option mostly with baked goods.

- Tofu provides a nutritious amount of protein in similar amounts as an egg would. Tofu is a great alternative for heavy egg recipes such as scrambled eggs, quiche and omelets.

Meat: Letting go of animal meats has never been easier. Companies are making so many products such as veggie meatballs, veggie bacon, veggie sausages, soy chicken patties and many more. If you would still like to use substitutes for your favorite recipes here are some alternatives:

- Tofu: with ½ cup of tofu packing a whopping 10 grams of protein this is a great meat alternative. Feel free to mix in some ground flax seeds to add some texture, since tofu's texture tends to be light and fluffy.

- Garbanzo beans contain as much as 12 grams of protein in a cup. They can easily be cooked, mashed and shaped into your favorite meals.

- Ground walnuts or almonds are perfect for when you need to add texture to any recipe, allowing for a more chewy and crunchy feel in every bite.

Honey: Some vegans that aren't very strict with their diet and will consume honey, but in this case I am offering you a wonderful vegan alternative as is:

- Agave syrup: This plant based syrup is sweeter than honey so a little goes a long way. It's a fantastic option for smoothies, tea, desserts and more.

- Maple syrup is lower in calories than honey. Ideally you will purchase a less processed maple syrup to enjoy its full flavor. Maple syrup is full of zinc, iron, and many other minerals.

Chocolate: If you've got a sweet tooth as I do, there is no way you could ever give up chocolate. Luckily you don't have to. There are many non-dairy vegan chocolates, powders, and even chocolate bars.

Ice Cream: With all the milk alternatives available, you can easily find or even make ice cream with a nut base, rice base, coconut base and more. You can even opt for a fruit sorbet sweetened with agave. Even the kids will love it!

Try it

Yes, you could just give up now and say there's no way you can do this. But if you're looking for a healthier body and lifestyle then at least try it.

Before you go on to say how hard this is going to be for you, think about all the benefits that will come from it. Nothing but good things will come from this change in your life.

Start small begin by minimizing grains, sugar and processed foods gradually and see how your body feels.

When I began I thought of how much I loved eating croissants, and cheese sandwiches, but began slowly pulling away from these foods. Pretty soon I noticed that I was no longer missing these foods and even noticed they did not sit well with me, I felt bloated and fatigued after eating them

Begin with 30 days of complete discipline. After 30 days your body will begin to adjust from fueling itself on carbs and sugar to using your stored fat for energy.

The closer you shift your diet to vegan principles, the quicker you will begin to see and feel the results. Let's get started!

Chapter 4
Clean and Organic

"You are what you eat- so don't be easy, fast cheap or fake." M. Allen

Think you will go far in any sport by just doing the training and ignoring what you eat? Think again!

The proper nutrition is the foundation of health and performance, and in order to achieve your full athletic potential you must tune up your diet. What you ingest will greatly affect how you look, feel and perform, yet most athletes make their nutrition secondary in their training. Your nutrition affects you in every way possible, from your skin, your thoughts, your strength and speed.

Food quality

Before we begin to focus on portions and calories let's focus on the quality of your food. I want you to think about the last time you went to the supermarket, what aisles did you visit, what did you place in your cart?

I will let you in a secret, the next time you go to the supermarket focus ninety percent of your shopping on the perimeter of the grocery store. Only venture down the aisles for a few select foods like nuts. If you realize the healthy foods are perishable therefore they are in the perimeters of the store. Unlike the aisles which are full of processed foods with ingredients you have no idea what they are and most of time can't even pronounce.

Healthy foods are perishable. They are organic plants and foods our bodies were built to consume. If a sugary cereal has a shelf life of several years, how good can eating that be for your body? It clearly has no organic material left, or it has been coated with enough chemicals to delay the decay. We now begin to wonder what effects those chemicals have on your body and mind. Many will say there is no evidence to sustain they do no harm, yet we know they do no good either.

Organic and Natural

Organic food has become a popular term lately. Years ago organic food was available only in health stores or in farmers markets, nowadays it has become widely available in many grocery markets.

What does organic mean? The term refers to the manner in which agricultural products are grown and processed.

In the beginning of farming all foods were organic. It was as simple as placing the seed in the ground and harvesting when ready. They were all grown free of pesticides and chemical fertilizers. Foods were minimally processed, unrefined and whole.

Today with the population growing, farming has taken a turn and tried to supply more and more with the help of pesticides and chemicals. This has made our foods not only deficient in nutrients, but also full of chemicals and toxins making it difficult for us to be healthy and well balanced.

In order to qualify as organic crops and livestock must be:

Organic crops must be grown in safe soil, have no modification or be genetically modified, and must remain separate from conventional food. Farmers are not allowed to use synthetic pesticides and petroleum or sewage based fertilizers.

Benefits of Eating Organic Food

- More nutrients. Several studies have shown that organically grown foods contain more nutrients than non-organic grown foods because the soil is sustained and nourished with healthy practices. The nitrogen that is found in composted soil is slowly released this way plants can grow at a normal rate, with their nutrients in balance.

- Better Taste. Many foods are now being modified to enhance their colors and achieve a more consistent shape. In return, the taste is not taken into account. Organic foods might not always be prettiest or shiniest, but they sure are the tastiest.

- Pesticide and chemical free. Research from the past few years demonstrate the negative effects of these toxins in our body such as cancer, asthma, brain function and more.

- Promote the local economy. Organic foods are quite often grown locally, visit your local market, you will probably get a better price and a fresher product.

- Organic Farming is better for the environment. These farms are sustainable, reduce pollution, conserve water and use less energy.

Cost vs. Health

This kind of grocery shopping will most likely be more expensive than you're used to. Fresh organic food costs more because it's real food. It will spoil quickly unlike processed foods which can be stored in boxes for months and still be edible somehow.

If you find buying fresh and organic to be too expensive for you can also opt for frozen vegan meats, fruits and vegetables as an option.

Every year the EWG Environmental Working Group releases a list of 12 foods that you should always whenever available buy organic. It has been estimated individuals can decrease their exposure by 80% if they change to organic when purchasing those foods. The group analyzes which foods contain the highest pesticide residue and call those 12 the dirty dozen. Each year some foods change, but over the past couple of years these are the foods that have been on the dirty dozen consistently.

1. Strawberries
2. Grapes
3. Celery
4. Peaches
5. Spinach
6. Potatoes
7. Cherries
8. Lettuce
9. Cucumbers
10. Blueberries
11. Sweet bell Peppers
12. Nectarines

You must decide for yourself if eating this way is worth the cost. Personally I try to make cuts in other areas of my budget, but I find my health more important than anything else. Of course the bag of Cheetos is cheap and easy, but I am not willing to eat that when I have better options available.

Many of these changes might seem extreme from your current way of life. But if you want to improve your health and performance these changes are necessary.

You can choose to eat cheap and fast now and pay for it later or spend a little more on healthier food now but enjoy a better life on the long term.

Chapter 5

Macronutrients

"Anyone can work out for an hour, but to control what goes on your plate for 23 hours… now that's hard work." Anonymous

Nutrition is the most important characteristic in order to achieve your goals. Consider your body a fine-tuned Lamborghini and your muscles the engine. If you don't supply your engine with the correct fuel during a competition you won't perform half as well as your fine-tuned body could.

Even in your day to day life your body requires the correct kind of nutrition. If you know you're overweight by 10 pounds and think it's not that much try strapping on a 10 pound vest and see how well you perform with it on. Yes, those extra pounds will definitely hinder your performance.

Nutrition is different for each individual, and as such this is an overview of recommendations designed to help you as you plan your nutritional requirements for competing, training or for day to day meals.

Protein

Protein is a very important component in an athlete's diet, after all your muscles are made of protein. Protein is essential is promoting fast muscle recovery after workouts and to ensure your muscles adapt fully in response to your training, in order words, you start toning that body.

They are often called the building blocks of the body. Protein consists of a combination of structures called amino acids that combine in several ways to help create muscles, bone, tendons, skin, hair, and other tissues. Athletes need protein to assist in repairing and rebuilding muscle that was broken down during exercise. It also helps to optimize carbohydrate storage in the form of glycogen.

There are many doubts in this area, many believe that eating more protein will make you gain weight. When you train your muscles need to be replenished which is why they need protein to rebuild and restructure.

Athletes require more protein than individuals who don't train. If a sedentary person were to consume the same amount of protein an athlete consumes, then surely all the unused protein would turn into fat and weight gain would occur.

As long as you're training the protein you consume will repair your muscles and help you stay toned and healthy.

Research has proven that the timing of protein intake plays an important role. Eating high quality protein within two hours after exercising enhances muscle healing and development.
The length and intensity of the exercise is also very important when it comes to protein requirements. Power training needs a higher level of protein intake than endurance training does because power is focusing more on building muscle.

General Requirements
Research has proved the adequate intake of protein for improved athletic performance as 0.6 to 0.9 grams of protein per pound of body weight or 1.4 to 2 grams per kilogram. For example a 160 pound athlete requires 102 to 146 grams of protein per day.

As we mentioned above the intensity and purpose of training also make a difference in daily protein intake. We will review three possibilities below, endurance training, strength training and training to reduce fat.

- Endurance Training

According to the intensity of the training we could estimate that when training at a light to moderate regimen you would need 0.5 to 0.8 grams of protein per pound of body weight. When training in a high intensity regimen 0.7 to 0.9 grams per pound of body weight are recommended.

- Strength Training

It's recommended that when you are focusing on strength training in an intense regimen to consume 0.6 to 0.9 grams of protein per pound of body weight or 1.5 to 2.0 grams per kilogram of body weight. This amount is ideal to optimize muscle mass, strength and physical performance.

- Reduce Body Fat

When you are focused on reducing body fat but maintain your lean muscle mass the recommended protein intakes can be as high as 1.0 to 1.5 grams of protein per pound of body weight. These numbers can increase even more if you are restricting your calorie intake. Your goal at this time would be to maintain your lean muscles while burning off fat.

Where to find protein

Some examples of foods that contain protein are soy, legumes, lentil, beans, nuts and several vegetables such as avocado, cauliflower, asparagus, broccoli and artichoke.

My top recommendation for protein sources for athletes are:

Almonds

Protein is also found in plant foods such as nuts. It does not offer as much protein as animal foods, but when it comes to plant foods almonds are an excellent choice. Two ounces of dry roasted and salted almonds contains twelve grams of protein. Almonds also provide vitamin E, Fiber and much more.

Soy

Most likely the best plant source of protein. It can be found in many different ways such as tofu, edamame, soy milk, soy burgers, and soy protein based powdered drink mixes.

Protein Powder Hemp, Chia and Pea Blend

The closest there is to a perfect protein source. Commonly found in a variety of powdered drink mixes, nutrition bars, and more. Many studies have found that intakes of protein powder accelerate post-training recovery and enhance muscle performance.

Lentils

They are and easy and tasty way to consume a high dose of protein. With only ½ cup you will add 9 grams of protein and almost 15 grams of fiber to your meal.

Quinoa

There are incredibly versatile in many recipes and pack 8 grams of protein per cup. It also contains nine essential amino acids our bodies need for repair and growth.

Chia Seeds

With an impressive 5 grams of protein in 2 tablespoons, this little seeds pack quite a punch. They're easy to sprinkle on smoothies, salads and desserts.

Carbohydrates

They are the most important source of energy for athletes. No matter what sport you play, carbs provide the energy that fuels muscle contractions. Once carbs are consumed, they breakdown into smaller sugars that get absorbed and used as energy. A steady supply of carbohydrate intake prevents protein from being used as energy. The body stores carbohydrates as glycogen in the muscles and liver, but its holding capacity is limited. When the fuel needs of an athlete are not met with the stored carbohydrate the consequences include fatigue, reduced ability to train hard, impaired thoughts, and a decrease in immune system function.

For these reasons, athletes should plan their carbohydrate intake around key training sessions and their day to day requirements with carbohydrates as an exercise fuel.

Your carbohydrate requirements depend on the fuel needed in your training and competition program. The exact amount is dependent on the frequency, duration and intensity of the activity. Since your activities will change every day your carbohydrate intake should fluctuate to reflect this. On days with high activity carbohydrate intake should be increased to match the increase in activity. This increase will allow your body to maximize your activity and promote recovery between sessions.

On the other hand on low or no training days carbohydrate intake should be decreased to reflect the decrease in activity. A smart way to regulate carbohydrate intake from day to day is to schedule foods that are carbohydrate rich at meals or snacks around important activity sessions. As the intensity of the sessions increase you should increase your carbohydrate intake before, during or after exercising. This not only helps to have the proper amount of carbohydrates, but also it improves the timing so it's best suited to fuel the session.

The following numbers are a good standard to go by:

Light Training: Low intensity. 3-5 grams per kilogram of body weight.

Moderate Training: Average activity for approximately 1 hour. 5-7 grams per kilogram of body weight.

Intense Training. High intensity activity for 1-3 hours per day. 6-10 grams per kilogram of body weight.

Extreme training. Very high intensity activity for more than 4 hours per day. 8-12 grams per kilogram of body weight.

Simple and Complex Carbohydrates

Carbohydrates are both simple and complex.

Simple carbohydrates have a smaller structure with only 1 or 2 sugar molecules. Some simple carbohydrates include sucrose, sugar found in candy, soda, juice. They are the fastest source of energy, as they are quickly digested, but only last for a short period of time. They tend to have little or no vitamins and minerals.

Complex carbohydrates are made of many sugar molecules looped together like a necklace. They are commonly rich in fiber, and health promoting. Complex carbohydrates are usually found in whole plant foods and, hence, are also often full of vitamins and minerals. Examples would be cassava, yam, white potato, green vegetables, peas, sweet potatoes, pumpkin and other vegetables.

My top 5 recommendation for carbohydrate sources for athletes are:

Sweet Potatoes

One of my favorite carbohydrates since it provides so many nutrients in each bite. They are very high in antioxidants and potassium which helps sooth sore muscles. One cup equals 27 grams of carbs.

Berries

You name it, strawberries, blueberries, blackberries, and other berries are among the most nutritious sources of carbohydrates. They are not the most concentrated source of carbohydrates with only 12grams in one cup but they are extremely rich in vitamins, minerals and phytonutrients.

Bananas

The most common snack for athletes is easy to digest and loaded with fast acting carbohydrates. Bananas are a great pre or post exercise snack with 31 grams of carbohydrates.

Chestnuts

They are a great snack that provides quite a bit of fiber, vitamin C and folic acid. Chestnuts can be served roasted, in soups, stuffing and many more ways. Compared to other nuts chestnuts provide less than one gram of fat per ounce.

Oranges

They are an excellent option instead of bananas. One orange alone contains all the daily vitamin C requirements. Opt for the fruit instead of the juice so you can enjoy the benefits of the fiber as well.

Healthy Fats

Contrary to popular belief eating fat does not make you fat. It's the kind of fat you choose to eat that can make you fat.

Fat is one of the 3 macronutrients together with protein and carbohydrates that supply calories to the body. Fat provides 9 calories per gram which is more than twice the number offered by protein or carbohydrates.

Fat is actually one of the critical nutrients for optimal health and is essential for the proper functioning on the body. Fats provide essential fatty acids not made by the body and must be attained from food.

Omega-3 and Omega-6 fatty acids are required for normal growth and development and for the standard functioning of the brain and nervous system. Fat is the main storage source for the body's extra calories. It fills the fat cells that help insulate the body and it is also an important energy source. Fat is a fuel source for low-level to modest exercise such as walking or jogging, and is very important for extended endurance trials that are at lower intensities. After the body has used up all the calories from the carbohydrates consumed which normally occurs in the first 20-30 minutes of exercise it begins to rely on the calories from fat.

While fat is easily deposited in the body and is calorie-dense, it also takes longer to breakdown and digest. It can take up to 6 hours to be converted into a usable form of energy. This would clearly identify fat unsuitable as a pre- exercise snack and is why we choose carbohydrates to fuel our activities.

When consuming, choose "good fats" such as polyunsaturated and monounsaturated fats which are found in nuts, seeds, canola and olive oils, flax seeds and avocados.

Do not eat foods with "bad fats" such as potato chips, ice cream or any solid fat. They contain trans fats and saturated fats. Too much of these have been linked to health problems such as obesity, high cholesterol, heart disease and poor athletic performance.

Fats should represent no more than 25% to 30% of your total calorie intake. High-fat foods must be avoided as they can cause uneasiness if eaten too close to the start of physical activity. No consumption of trans fats and saturated fats. Emphasize healthy fats that are found in avocados, canola oil, soy, and nuts.

My top recommendations for fat sources for athletes are:

Flaxseed oil

We often cook with oils, and use oil in our salads and day to day meals, why not use oil that includes many of the same benefits as fish oil including a high level of Omega 3s. It's important to note that consuming flaxseeds alone we will not intake the same amount of omega 3s, flaxseeds must be ground up to release its fat content.

Avocados

Avocados are high in fat, but most of the fat in an avocado is in fact monounsaturated which is the heart-healthy kind that helps lower bad cholesterol. They make an excellent substitution for butter or cream cheese when needed.

Nuts

Walnuts, almonds, sunflower seeds, pistachios and pumpkin seeds are all very special nuts. They contain nutrients such as selenium, lutein, and are very high in vitamin E. Many of them are high in Omega 3 or Omega 6, they provide a good amount of fiber and are great for on the go snacks.

Chapter 6

Micronutrients

"You are given the opportunity to nourish your body with every bite and sip you take." M. Correa

Vitamins are vital elements that must be consumed because the body does not produce them by itself. They are essential to maintain healthy and balanced body functions.

Fruits and vegetables contain vitamins, minerals and antioxidants that are essential to maintaining a healthy and balanced diet. Examples are: Oranges, a great source for vitamin c, bananas for potassium, and carrots for beta carotene.

Two important minerals to consider in athletes are Calcium and Iron. Calcium helps build stronger bones, which decreases the chance of them breaking under stress or heavy activity. You can find calcium in many dairy products, such as milk, yogurt, and cheese. Also include dark, green leafy vegetables and calcium-fortified products, like orange juice as good sources of calcium.

Now we'll go into several important vitamins and minerals and better understand how they help us and where we can find them.

Vitamin A

Well known for proper vision development, it also has many other benefits. It maintains red and white blood cell production and activity. Promotes a healthy immune system, and keep skin healthy.

An optimal daily intake for a male would be 900 micrograms and for a female would be 700 micrograms.

Good sources of Vitamin A are squash, sweet potato, carrots, kale, apricot, peaches, cantaloupe, papaya, and mango.

In order to reach your optimal daily intake these foods contain a good amount of Vitamin A. It's important to remember that many vegetables loose many vitamins and nutrients when cooked.

Kale ½ cup = 443 mcg

Carrots ½ cup = 538 mcg

Cantaloupe ½ melon = 467 mcg

Spinach ½ cup = 573 mcg

Sweet Potato ½ cup = 961 mcg

Vitamin C

Vitamin C is essential for the biosynthesis of collagen. Collagen is the main protein used as connective tissue in the body. Collagen is especially important for healthy joints, ligaments, and bones. Other benefits of vitamin C include a boost in the immune system, supports in wound healing and improves brain function.

An optimal daily intake for a male or female would be 45 to 75 micrograms.

Good sources of Vitamin C are citrus fruits, leafy greens, peppers, and cauliflower.

In order to reach your optimal daily these foods contain a good amount of Vitamin C.

Red pepper raw ½ cup = 95 mcg

Orange juice ¾ cup = 93 mcg

Broccoli cooked ½ cup = 51 mcg

Kiwi fruit = 64 mcg

Strawberries ½ cup = 49 mcg

Vitamin D

Vitamin D is vital for proper calcium metabolism. Bone density is linked directly to this vitamin, as well as a good nervous system function and immunity.

This vitamin is a special one, it allows your body to manufacture Vitamin D when you get sunlight on your skin. No need to bask in the sunlight, no more than few minutes a day are required.

Vitamin D is not easily found in food in nature, which is why many products are now fortified with this Vitamin such as soy milk and orange juice.

An optimal daily intake for a male or female would be 15 mcg.

Vitamin E

Vitamin E is also called the excellent vitamin. It pertains to a family of eight antioxidants and as such protects our bodies from damage. Constantly battling free radicals protects essential lipids and maintains the balance of cell membranes. Naturally an anti-inflammatory, it aids in muscle wellness.

An optimal daily intake for a male or female would be15 micrograms.

Good sources of Vitamin E are nuts, seeds, avocado, wheat grains, and oils.

In order to reach your optimal daily these foods contain a good amount of Vitamin E.

Wheat germ oil 1 tablespoon = 20 mcg

Sunflower seeds 1 ounce = 7.4 mcg

Peanut butter 2 tablespoons = 2.9 mcg

Almonds roasted 1 ounce = 6.8 mcg

Vitamin K

The K in vitamin K is from German origin for "Koagulation" which means coagulation in German. This vitamin is essential for coagulation in our bodies. Deficiencies are visible with easy bruising, nosebleeds, and heavy menstrual periods.

An optimal daily intake for a male would be 80 mcg or female would be 65 micrograms.

Vitamin K is readily available in many foods we eat day to day, but is especially concentrated in leafy greens.

Kale ½ cup = 531 mcg

Spinach ½ cup = 444 mcg

Broccoli 1 cup = 220 mcg

Swiss Chard 1 cup = 290 mcg

Minerals

Minerals are nutrients your body requires to function properly. They are consumed mostly in animal and plant form. Without these minerals we would be prone to illness, and a lack of performance.

Zinc

Zinc is a trace element that is found in natural foods, fortified foods and as a dietary supplement. It aids in the breakdown of protein, fat and carbohydrates. It also assists in wound healing and immune wellbeing. Zinc deficiency is dangerous because it supports proper growth and development of the body.

An optimal daily intake for a male and female would be 8 to 11 micrograms.

Zinc is readily available in many foods we eat day to day such as:

Oatmeal cooked 1 cup = 2.3 mg

Sunflower seeds roasted ¼ cup = 1.7 mg

Lentils cooked ½ cup = 1.3 mg

Potassium

This mineral and electrolyte is important enough to make our heart beat. Yes, its functions include the transmission of nervous system signals, muscle movement, and a steady heartbeat. Potassium also lowers blood pressure and also helps our bones.

This mineral is essential to any athlete any deficiency leads to muscle cramping, vomiting and fatigue.

An optimal daily intake for a male and female would be approximately 2000 mg.

Many sports drinks include potassium, and we often see athletes eating a banana or two which also contains potassium. But these foods are also good sources:

Plums ½ cup = 637 mg

Baked Potatoes = 926 mg

Raisins ½ cup = 598 mg

Banana = 422 mg

Iron

Iron is essential for growth, development, synthesis of several hormones, and normal functioning. But it's most important function is to help hemoglobin and myoglobin (components of red blood cells and muscles) bring oxygen to all the cells that require it.

An optimal daily intake for a male would be 8 mg. and female would be 15 mg.

The following are excellent sources of iron:

Cooked lentils ½ cup = 3.30 mg

Spinach boiled ½ cup = 3 mg

Tofu ½ cup = 3 mg

Calcium

Calcium is probably the most talked about mineral and the most abundant mineral in our bodies.

Calcium is crucial for the wellbeing of bones, teeth, and muscle contraction. A deficiency in this mineral will cause poor teeth and brittle bones.

An optimal daily intake for a male and female would be 1300 mg.

Kale raw 1 cup = 100 mg

Broccoli boiled 1 cup = 62 mg

Collards boiled 1 cup = 266 mg

White beans boiled 1 cup = 161

Magnesium

Magnesium is a mineral that collaborates with calcium to help with proper muscle contraction, energy metabolism, blood clotting, and building healthy teeth and bones.

Magnesium is widely available in plants and animal foods. An optimal daily intake for an male would be 240-400 mg or female would be 250-350 mg

Good sources of magnesium are:

Brazil nuts 1 ounce = 107 mg

Pumpkin 1 ounce = 151 mg

Banana = 44 mg

Dietary Supplements

As competitors, athletes are looking to for ways to achieve their peak performance. You can complete your daily requirements your body needs with a proper diet, however many athletes turn to supplements because they believe it's a better way to optimize their health and performance. It's important to realize there is no "super pill" that can compensate for a poor diet. In order to maintain your body healthy and at its peak a balanced diet is required. But to avoid any deficiency in vitamins and minerals a dietary supplement is recommended. Supplements are meant to do exactly what their name says, supplements your regular food intake. These are not a substitute for a healthy diet or to cure any medical conditions. We would consider them as a backup, to complete the requirements of any missing vitamins or minerals in our diet.

Some supplements will definitely help you make faster improvements in your strength and composition, but before even thinking about that focus on your diet. If what you eat is not right then no supplement can help you achieve your goals.

Many vegan supplements are easily available in health stores pharmacies, supermarkets or vitamin stores. Always look at the ingredient list not all supplements are made the same, make sure you're choosing natural and organic when purchasing.

It's also important to keep in mind what exactly you're goals are before administering these supplements. Please be mindful and consult with your doctor before taking any supplements.

Extra tips

Include foods rich in iron in your diet, like vegan meat, dried beans, and fortified cereals. With a decreased iron diet, energy levels in athletes decrease. Females who have their menstrual cycle lose iron every month. Another way many minerals are lost is through their sweat.

Eat more Vegetables and Fruits

Not only are they packed with vitamins, minerals and phytonutrients most fruits and vegetables also contain a great sum of fiber and water. Studies have demonstrated we have a tendency to consume a consistent amount of food each day, regardless of the amount of calories contained. Water and fiber enhance the volume of foods without increasing calories. So you would be eating the same volume of food, but now with less calories and healthier.

An easy way to increase your fruit and vegetable intake is to consider each meal a **colorful one**. Aim for at least 4 or more colors with each meal, such as: carrots (orange) 1, spinach (green) 2, tomato (red) 3, potato (white) 4, lentils (brown) 5. The more colors, the more nutrients your body is acquiring.

Avoid at all times

We must have the same discipline in training as we do in our nutrition. Many of the following foods can be eaten on a rare occasion, but they should not be considered a snack or part of an everyday diet.

Foods like chips, Cheetos, sweets, cakes, cookies, carbonated sodas, fast foods, artificial colors, high fructose corn syrup, preservatives and empty calorie snacks. They will hinder performance and decrease overall good health.

Remember: **When you think you're done training, you're not done training, at least not until you've put some nutrients back into your body.**

Just as important as your workout is what you do as soon as you finish your workout. If you forget to nourish your body, you'll never get the full worth out of all the work you just put in… and what a waste that would be.

Your best performance simply won't happen if you lose focus on your body's needs for nutrients. Give your body what it needs immediately after exercising, when it's most receptive to replenishment, and it will respond wonderfully.

Chapter 7

Vegan Smoothies

I love the concept of going to the kitchen and using just one machine to get tons of nutrients in each sip I take. This is the beauty of blending, you can add tons of nutrients, colors and tastes to your diet. A super packed nutritious smoothie in just a few minutes, perfect for a quick boost to your diet.

Smoothies are all the hype at the moment, but not all of them are as healthy as they say. Many of them are filled with enough sugar for an entire day's worth. Others lack protein or fiber.

Protein is very important for athletes for many reasons but principally for its capability to repair muscles, aid in muscle regrowth and keep your metabolism working properly.

While vegan protein powders are very convenient, they are not always budget friendly or have all the nutrients and fiber whole foods have.

These are some of the best alternatives to protein powders to add some protein to your smoothie:

Raw hulled Hemps seeds

By simply adding 3 tablespoons of hemp seed you will be increasing 13 grams of healthy protein to your smoothie. Hemp seeds are also high in iron, magnesium, Vitamin E and K.

Raw Pumpkin seeds

These are one of the most alkaline seeds you can eat. Pumpkin seeds are rich in magnesium, potassium, iron and protein. They contain as much as 5 grams of protein per ¼ cup.

Raw Quinoa

A very well-known superfood with incredible properties, even N.A.S.A. has praised this superfood that has been known to grow even in outer space. Only 100 grams of quinoa contains 14 grams of protein.

Almond Butter

Feel free to add raw almonds or almond butter, make sure the almond butter contains no added oils or salt. 2 tablespoons of almond butter lends 7-8 grams of protein. Almonds are also great sources of Vitamin E, magnesium, potassium and fiber.

Chia Seeds

These are one of my favorite seeds, they tend to puff up in liquid and give a nice creamy taste to any smoothie. An amazing source of energy, nutrients and protein with ¼ cup of chia seeds providing 10 grams of protein.

Spirulina

Green goodness packed in every teaspoon with 4 grams of protein in every teaspoon.

Nuts, and seeds tend to be a great addition to any smoothie. You can easily combine and match any of these to add more protein to your smoothies.

Ready, set, get your blenders out and try a whole explosion of nutrients and protein in your next level smoothie!

Chapter 8

Recipes

"You don't have to cook fancy or complicated masterpieces – just good food from fresh ingredients." Julia Child

These are several of my favorite recipes that I am sharing with you, feel free to adapt and expand these recipes with other vegan foods. Be creative with your meals, mix and match foods. Think of your favorite meals and combine them into something great. Try new foods you've never tried before, you might be surprised.

Nature provides us with so much variety with textures, flavors and colors, we are extremely lucky to be able to enjoy it all.

In this chapter you will find a total of 50 vegan protein smoothie recipes. Feel free to add even more protein to these smoothie by adding some of the nuts, seeds and ingredients we mentioned in our previous chapter.

I hope you enjoy them all!

1. Tomato protein shake:

Ingredients:

1 glass of rice milk

¼ tsp of cinnamon

1 small tomato

1 grated carrot

1 tsp of vegan cane sugar

Preparation:

Wash and cut tomato into small cubes. Peel and grate the carrot. You want to cut the carrot into thin strips. Mix the ingredients in a blender and keep in the refrigerator for about 20 minutes before serving.

2. Vegetable protein shake

Ingredients:

1 cup of chopped broccoli

Half bunch of fresh spinach

½ cup of vegan Greek yogurt

1 tbsp of agave syrup

Few mint leaves, chopped

¼ cup of water

Preparation:

Wash the vegetables and put into a blender. Put some ice cubes and blend together until smooth mixture.

3. Mixed fruits and vegetables protein shake

Ingredients:

1 cup of mixed blueberries, raspberries, blackberries and strawberries

½ cup of chopped baby spinach

¼ cup of ground almonds

½ cup of cashew cream

1.5 glass of water

Preparation:

Wash the baby spinach and put it in a blender. Mix cashew cream with almonds, add water and put in a blender. Add berries and mix for few minutes. Serve cold.

4. Melon protein shake

Ingredients:

1 slice of melon

¼ cup of fresh strawberries

¼ of banana

½ tsp of cinnamon

¼ cup of chopped walnuts

1 tbsp of brown sugar

1 cup of water

Preparation:

Mix ingredients in a blender and sprinkle with cinnamon. Keep in the refrigerator and serve cold.

5. Strawberry protein shake:

Ingredients:

1 cup of strawberries

½ cup of almond milk

1 tbsp of chia seeds

1 tbsp of agave syrup

Preparation:

Mix the ingredients in a blender for few minutes. Leave it in the refrigerator for few minutes and serve cold. You can add some ice cubes in it.

6. Vanilla protein shake

Ingredients:

1 glass of flax milk

½ glass of water

1 tsp of vanilla extract

1 tsp of minced vanilla

1 tbsp of hemp seeds, minced

¼ tsp of cinnamon

2 tsp of turbinado sugar

Preparation:

Mix the flax milk with water and boil on a low temperature. Add minced vanilla and vanilla extract. Stir well and let it boil for about a minute. Remove from the heat and allow it to cool. Mix with other ingredients in a blender for few minutes. Serve cold.

7. Broccoli protein shake

Ingredients:

1 cup of cooked or raw broccoli

1 glass of water

½ cup of oat milk

1 cup of goji berries

1 tbsp of pumpkin seeds

1 tbsp of turbinado sugar

1 tsp of agave syrup

Preparation:

Mix the ingredients in a blender for few minutes. Serve this healthy drink cold.

8. Coffee protein shake

Ingredients:

1 cup of unsweetened chilled coffee

½ cup of macadamia nut milk

2 macadamia nuts, minced

2 tsp of vanilla extract

2 tsp of brown sugar

1 tbsp of vegan Greek yogurt

cinnamon (optional)

Preparation:

Combine all the ingredients in a blender. Mix well for about 30 seconds. Drink cold. You can add some cinnamon on top, but this is optional. Keep this protein shake in the refrigerator, or you can even freeze it for later use.

9. Apple and orange protein shake

Ingredients:

1 small apple

1 small orange

½ glass of water

1 tsp of brown sugar

1 tbsp of agave nectar

1 tbsp of almonds, minced

Preparation:

Put all the ingredients in a blender for few minutes. Drink cold.

10. Fruit protein shake

Ingredients:

1 cup of fresh blueberries

1 banana

1 tbsp of applesauce

1 Indian nut

½ tsp of cinnamon

½ glass of rice milk

1 tbsp of agave syrup

Preparation:

Peel the banana and cut into small pieces. Combine agave syrup with applesauce and rice milk and boil briefly. Allow it to cool for a while. Mix the ingredients in a blender for about 30 seconds. Sprinkle with cinnamon and serve cold.

11.   Oatmeal protein shake

Ingredients:

½ cups of oatmeal

1 cup of almond milk

1 tbsp of almonds, minced

¼ cup of water

1 tsp of vanilla extract

½ banana, sliced

Preparation:

This recipe takes only few minutes to prepare and it is super tasty. All you want to do is combine the ingredients in a blender and mix until smooth mixture for about 30-40 seconds. Leave in the refrigerator for 30 minutes. You can sprinkle some cinnamon on top.

12.   Peppermint protein shake

Ingredients:

2 cups of hemp milk

1 tsp of cocoa powder, organic

1 tbsp of grated almonds

1 tbsp of almond cream

½ tsp of peppermint extract

Preparation:

Boil the hemp milk on a low temperature. Add peppermint extract and cocoa powder. Stir well for 2-3 minutes. Remove from the heat and allow it to cool for about 30 minutes. Combine with the grated almonds and almond cream. Put in a blender for about 30 seconds. Serve cold.

13.   Flaxseed oil protein shake

Ingredients:

½ cup of water

½ cup of cashew milk

1 tbsp of grated walnuts

1 tbsp of goji berries

1 tbsp of flaxseed oil

1 tsp of vanilla extract

1 tbsp of brown sugar

Preparation:

Mix the ingredients in a blender for about 40 seconds, or until smooth mixture. Keep in the refrigerator and serve cold.

14.   Cinnamon protein shake

Ingredients:

1 cup of hazelnut milk

1 tsp of cocoa powder

1 tbsp of raisins

1 tbsp of pumpkin seeds

¼ tsp of cinnamon

Preparation:

Mix in a blender until smooth mixture. Serve with ice cubes. You can sprinkle some more cinnamon on top before serving.

15.   Almond protein shake

Ingredients:

1 cup of almond milk

½ cup of water

1 tbsp of ground flax meal

1 tbsp of grated almonds

1 tbsp of agave nectar

½ cup of oatmeal

Preparation:

Combine the ground flax meal with 3 tbsp of water and mix well. Combine with other ingredients and mix in a blender for 30-40 seconds. Allow it to cool in the refrigerator. Serve cold.

16. Banana protein shake

Ingredients:

1 large banana

1 cup of oat milk

½ cup of water

1 tbsp of flax seeds

1 tbsp macadamia nut, minced

1 tsp of vanilla extract

1 tbsp of agave syrup

Preparation:

Peel and chop banana into small cubes. Combine with other ingredients in a blender and mix for 30 seconds, until smooth mixture. Keep in the refrigerator and serve cold.

17.   Bran flakes protein shake

Ingredients:

1 cup of coconut milk

½ cup of water

½ cup of bran flakes

1 tbsp of pumpkin seeds

1 tbsp of hazelnuts, ground

1 tbsp of brown sugar

1 tbsp of maple syrup

1 tsp of cocoa

Preparation:

Mix in a blender for 30-40 seconds, or until smooth mixture. You can add some cinnamon, but this is optional. Allow it to cool in the refrigerator for about an hour. Serve cold.

18.   Fresh mix protein shake

Ingredients:

½ cup of wild berries, fresh

½ cup of fresh wild berries juice

½ cup of water

1 tsp of blackberry extract

½ cup of pistachios, ground

1 tbsp of maple syrup

1 tbsp of agave sauce

1 handful of ice cubes

Preparation:

This high protein recipe will take less than 5 minutes to prepare. Combine the ingredients and mix in a blender for about 30 seconds. Serve cold.

19.   Walnuts protein shake

Ingredients:

1 cup of coconut milk

½ cup of grated walnuts

½ cup of finely chopped spinach

1 tbsp of agave syrup

2 tbsp of brown sugar

1 tsp of walnut extract

Preparation:

Combine the ingredients in a blender and mix for 30-40 seconds. Add some ice cubes before serving.

20. Vegan Greek yogurt protein shake

Ingredients:

1 cup of vegan Greek yogurt

1 tbsp of cashew cream

1 tbsp of almond cream

¼ cup of almond milk

1 tsp of almond butter

1 tbsp of brown sugar

¼ tsp of cinnamon

Preparation:

Combine the milk, almond butter, almond cream and brown sugar in a saucepan. Stir well and allow it to boil, on a low temperature for about 2 minutes. Remove from the heat and cool for 15 minutes. Pour the mixture in a blender and add other ingredients. Mix well for 30-40 seconds and keep in the refrigerator to cool.

21. Protein shake with coconut flakes

Ingredients:

1 cup of coconut milk

½ cup of water

½ cup of coconut flakes

1 tbsp of vegan Greek yogurt

3 tbsp of hazelnut cream

1 tsp of vanilla extract

1 tbsp of brown sugar

Preparation:

Combine the ingredients in a blender and mix until smooth mixture. Serve cold.

22.   Peanut butter protein shake

Ingredients:

1 cup of rice milk

¼ cup of finely chopped peanuts

1 tbsp of peanut butter

1 tbsp of brown sugar

1 tbsp of goji berries

1 small green apple

Preparation:

Peel and chop the apple into thin slices. Use a saucepan to melt the peanut butter on a low temperature. Add brown sugar and stir well for 30 seconds. Remove from the heat and allow it to cool. Meanwhile, mix the other ingredients in a blender, add peanut and sugar and mix well for 30-40 seconds. Keep in the refrigerator for at least 30 minutes to cool.

23.   Energy protein shake

Ingredients:

1 tbsp of grated almonds

1 tbsp of grated walnuts

1 tbsp of grated macadamia nuts

1 cup of strawberries

1 medium banana

1 glass of fresh orange juice

1 glass of water

2 tbsp of applesauce

1 tbsp of brown sugar

Preparation:

This protein shake is very easy to prepare. Simply combine the ingredients in a blender and mix well for 40 seconds. Cool well before serving.

24.   Pistachio protein shake

Ingredients:

1 cup of hemp milk

¼ cup of finely chopped pistachios

1 tbsp of peanut butter

1 tbsp of flax seeds, ground

1 tbsp of agave syrup

1 handful of ice

Preparation:

Mix the ingredients in a blender until smooth mixture.

25.   Almond butter protein shake

Ingredients:

1 cup of almond milk

½ cup of water

½ cup of oatmeal

1 tbsp of turbinado sugar

2 tbsp of almond butter

1 tsp of almond extract

¼ cup of hazelnut milk

Preparation:

Boil the almond milk on a low temperature. Add almond extract, almond butter and brown sugar. Stir well and allow it to boil for 30-40 seconds. Remove from the heat and cool. Combine with other ingredients in a blender and mix well for 30 seconds. Serve cold.

26.   Green apple protein shake

Ingredients:

1 green apple

½ cup of agave syrup

1 glass of fresh apple juice

1 tbsp of grated walnuts

¼ tsp of cinnamon

Preparation:

Peel and cut the apple into thin slices. Mix with other ingredients in a blender for 30-40 seconds. Serve with ice cubes.

27.   Applesauce and banana protein shake

Ingredients:

1 cup of rice milk

1 medium banana

¼ cup of applesauce

1 tsp of banana extract

1 tbsp of vegan Greek yogurt

1 tbsp of almond cream

Preparation:

Peel and chop banana into small cubes. Mix with other ingredients in a blender for 30-40 seconds and allow it to cool in the refrigerator for about an hour. Serve cold.

28.   Mixed nuts protein shake

Ingredients:

1 tsp of grated almonds

1 tsp of grated walnuts

1 tsp of grated hazelnuts

1 tsp of grated macadamia nuts

1 glass of fresh orange juice

1 tbsp of agave syrup

1 tbsp of vegan orange ice cream

1 handful of ice cubes

Preparation:

Mix the ingredients in a blender for 30-40 seconds.

29.   Pineapple protein shake

Ingredients:

3 thick pineapple slices

1 cup of fresh pineapple juice

1 tbsp of macadamia nuts, ground

1 tbsp of walnuts, ground

2 tbsp of agave syrup

1 tbsp of brown sugar

1 tsp of pineapple extract

2 cherries for decoration

Preparation:

Peel the pineapple slices. Chop into small pieces. Mix with other ingredients in a blender for 30-40 seconds. Serve with ice and cherries on top.

30.   Exotic protein shake

Ingredients:

1 cup of coconut milk

½ banana

½ cup of chopped pineapple

1 tbsp of flax seeds

1 tbsp of pumpkin seeds

1 tsp of coconut extract

2 tbsp of almond cream

2 tbsp of brown sugar

Preparation:

Combine the ingredients in a blender for 30-40 seconds and mix well until smooth mixture. Serve with some ice cubes.

31.   Peach and cream protein shake

Ingredients:

1 medium pitted peach

1 glass of almond milk

1 tbsp of maple syrup

1 tbsp of vegan Greek yogurt

1 tsp of peach extract

1 tbsp of brown sugar

1 tsp of pumpkin seeds

1 handful of ice

Preparation:

Cut the peach into small pieces. Mix with other ingredients in a blender until smooth mixture.

32. Greek vanilla protein shake

Ingredients:

1 cup of vegan Greek vanilla yogurt

1 cup of almond milk

1 tbsp of grated macadamia nuts

1 medium banana

½ cup of strawberries

1 tsp of vanilla extract

Preparation:

Peel the banana and cut into small cubes.
Combine with the other ingredients in a
blender and mix until smooth mixture, about
30-40 seconds. You can sprinkle some vanilla
powder on top, but this is optional. Serve cold.

33.   Plum power shake

Ingredients:

3 ripe plums, pitted

1 cup of rice milk

½ cup of walnuts, ground

¼ cup of agave syrup

Preparation:

Mix the ingredients in a blender for 30-40 seconds. Serve cold.

34.   Lemon protein shake

Ingredients:

1 glass of fresh lemonade, without sugar

1 tbsp of lemon zest

2 tbsp of brown sugar

½ cup of cashew cream

1 tbsp of peanuts

1 tbsp of vanilla extract

1 tbsp of grated oat crackers

Preparation:

Put the ingredients into a blender and blend until you get a creamy consistency. Pour it in a glass and sprinkle with grated oat crackers. Serve cold.

35.   Caramel protein shake

Ingredients:

1 cup of hazelnut milk

½ cup of brown sugar

½ tsp of cinnamon

1 tsp of chocolate extract

1 tbsp of grated almonds

1 tbsp of Brazil nuts, minced

1 medium pear, chopped into small pieces

2 tbsp of vegan Greek yogurt

Preparation:

Use a saucepan to melt the sugar on a low temperature. Slowly add the hazelnut milk and stir well for about a minute. Your sugar will become a nice caramel. Remove from the heat and allow it to cool for a while. Meanwhile cut a pear into small pieces, combine with other ingredients in a blender, add caramel and blend for about 40 seconds. Pour the protein shake into a glass, sprinkle with cinnamon and add some ice cubes.

36.   Hazelnuts protein shake

Ingredients:

1 cup of hazelnut milk

½ cup of vegan chocolate Greek yogurt

1 tsp of cocoa powder

2 tbsp of grated hazelnuts

1 tbsp of apricot seeds

1 tbsp of pecans, ground

1 tbsp of brown sugar

1 tbsp of agave syrup

Preparation:

Combine the ingredients in a blender and mix until creamy mixture. Allow it to cool in the refrigerator for about 30 minutes.

37. Chocolate and coffee protein shake

Ingredients:

1 cup of strong black coffee, without sugar

½ cup of almond cream

3 tbsp of vegan Greek yogurt

1 tbsp of brown sugar

1 tsp of cocoa

¼ cup of grated dark chocolate (80% of cocoa, vegan)

1 tbsp of grated hazelnuts

Preparation:

Mix the ingredients in a blender for 30-40 seconds. Keep in the refrigerator and serve with ice cubes. Sprinkle some grated hazelnuts on top.

38.　　Cherry protein shake

Ingredients:

1 cup of fresh cherry juice, without sugar

1 cup of cherries

½ cup of hazelnuts

1 tbsp of chia seeds

1 tsp of cherry extract

1 tbsp of brown sugar

1 handful of ice

Preparation:

You just need to mix the ingredients in a blender for 30 seconds. Serve cold.

39.　　Mango protein shake

Ingredients:

1 cup of chopped mango

½ cup of oatmeal

1 tsp of pumpkin seeds

1 tsp of almond butter

1 cup of almond milk

1 tbsp of banana sauce

2 tbsp of brown sugar

Preparation:

Combine the ingredients and blend until incorporated. Top with some mango extract powder, but this is optional. Serve cold.

40.   Forest pleasure protein shake

Ingredients:

1 cup of fresh apple juice

½ cup of water

½ medium green apple

½ medium carrot

½ small peach

½ cup of mixed forest berries (raspberries, strawberries, blackberries)

½ cup of almonds, minced

1 tbsp of hemp seeds

1 tbsp of agave syrup

Preparation:

Mix in a blender until smooth mixture. Allow it to cool in the refrigerator for a while.

41.   Ginger protein shake

Ingredients:

1 medium banana

1 cup of cashew milk

1 cup of finely chopped spinach

1 tsp of grated ginger

¼ cup of hemp seeds

1 tsp of lemon juice

2 tbsp of maple syrup

Preparation:

Combine the maple syrup with lemon juice and grated ginger. Mix with other ingredients in a blender for about 30 seconds, until foamy mixture.

42.   Papaya protein shake

Ingredients:

1 cup of papaya puree

½ cup of oatmeal

1 cup of rice milk

½ cup of water

1 tbsp of goji berries

1 tbsp of agave syrup

2 tbsp of brown sugar

1 tbsp of chia seeds

1 tbsp of pumpkin seeds

Preparation:

Combine the ingredients in a blender and mix well until smooth mixture. Serve with some ice cubes.

43.   Blueberries protein shake

Ingredients:

1 cup of almond milk

1 cup of blueberries

1 tbsp of brown sugar

1 tsp of mint extract

1 tbsp of grated almonds

Preparation:

This is very simple to prepare. This protein shake is very refreshing and it only takes about 2-3 minutes to prepare it. Just mix the ingredients in a blender for 30 seconds and serve with ice cubes.

44.   Pumpkin pie protein shake

Ingredients:

1 cup of pumpkin puree

1 cup of rice milk

1 tbsp of turbinado sugar

1 tbsp of banana sauce, organic

1 medium banana

1 small green apple

2 tbsp of ground walnuts

1 tbsp of flax seeds

1 tsp of cinnamon

Preparation:

Peel and grate the apple. Cut banana into small pieces and combine the ingredients in a blender for 30-40 seconds. Sprinkle some cinnamon on top and leave in the refrigerator to cool for a while.

45.   Raspberries and cream protein shake

Ingredients:

1 cup of frozen raspberries

½ cup of almond cream

½ cup of vegan raspberries ice cream

1 tbsp of chia seeds

1 tbsp of grated hazelnuts

1 cup of water

1 tbsp of agave syrup

Preparation:

Mix the ingredients in a blender for 30-40 seconds. Drink cold.

46.   Chocolate and walnuts protein shake

Ingredients:

1 glass of hemp milk

½ cup of water

½ cup of grated walnuts

¼ cup of grated dark chocolate (80% of cocoa, vegan)

1 tbsp of agave cream

1 tbsp of flax seeds

1 tbsp of chia seeds

1 tbsp of vegan cane sugar

Preparation:

Mix the ingredients in a blender until smooth mixture. Leave in the refrigerator for about 30 minutes to cool. Serve with some cinnamon on top (optional).

47.   Macadamian nuts protein shake

Ingredients:

1 cup of almond milk

½ cup of water

1 tsp of almond butter

¼ cup of grated macadamia nuts

1 tbsp of applesauce

2 tbsp of turbinado sugar

Preparation:

Combine with other ingredients in a blender and mix well for about 30-40 seconds, or until smooth mixture. Serve cold.

48.   Light protein shake

Ingredients:

1 cup of water

1 cup of finely chopped spinach

1 tbsp of almond cream

½ cup of vegan Greek yogurt

1 tbsp of brown sugar

Orange extract (optional)

Preparation:

Combine all the ingredients in a blender for about 30-40 seconds. Allow it to cool in the refrigerator. It tastes great with few drops of orange extract, but this is optional.

49.   Almond milk protein shake

Ingredients:

1 cup of almond milk

1 medium banana

1 tbsp of almond cream

1 macadamia nut

1 Brazil nut

1 tbsp of maple syrup

Preparation:

Mix the ingredients in a blender until smooth mixture. Serve cold.

50.   Coconut protein shake

Ingredients:

1 cup of coconut milk

1 tsp of coconut extract

½ cup of chopped pineapple

1 tbsp of grated walnuts

1 tbsp of minced chia seeds

1 tbsp of brown sugar

Preparation:

Mix the ingredients in a blender for about 30-40 second. Serve with ice.

22110089R00071

Printed in Great Britain
by Amazon